TOP 10 YOGA POSES FOR BEGINNERS

Jessica Cota

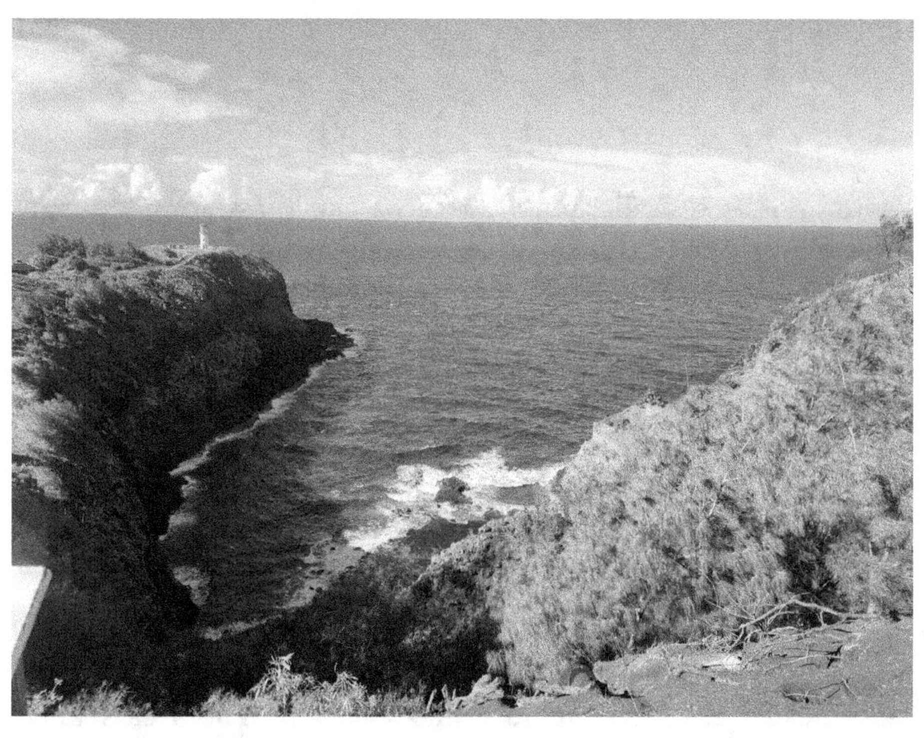

"Don't worry about anything; instead, pray about everything. Tell
God what you need, and thank Him for all He has done"
Philippians 4:6

Chapter 1

Mountain Pose (Tadasana)

Mountain Pose (Tadasana) is one of the most foundational yoga poses, perfect for beginners looking to establish balance, alignment, and mindfulness in their practice. Though it may appear simple, this pose is incredibly powerful in teaching body awareness and proper posture. To begin, stand tall with your feet together or hip-width apart, depending on your balance and comfort level. Ground your feet into the mat, ensuring your weight is distributed evenly across the soles of your feet. Engage your thigh muscles by gently lifting your kneecaps, and allow your tailbone to drop slightly as you engage your core.

As you move into the upper body, lengthen your spine by imagining a string gently pulling you upwards from the top of your head. Let your shoulders relax away from your ears, and keep your arms by your sides with your palms facing forward. Spread your fingers and keep them active, but without tension. Keep your chin parallel to the ground, and gently tuck it to lengthen the back of your neck. Throughout the pose, maintain a calm, steady breath, which helps you connect mind and body as you stand in stillness.

Mountain Pose serves as a great opportunity to cultivate mindfulness and focus. By paying attention to your posture and breath, you are practicing staying present in the moment. For beginners, this can be a valuable introduction to the meditative aspects of yoga. Over time, this pose strengthens your sense of balance and improves your body alignment, which can help reduce everyday tension in areas like the lower back, shoulders, and neck.

Physically, Mountain Pose helps build strength and stability in your legs, ankles, and feet. It encourages proper alignment throughout the body, which can improve posture and reduce the risk of injury. When practiced regularly, this pose can also enhance your awareness of how you carry yourself in your daily life, helping you walk and stand with more confidence and ease. Additionally, it promotes core engagement, which supports the spine and can improve overall body control.

Mentally, Tadasana fosters a sense of grounding and calm. The stillness of the pose allows you to focus inward, bringing attention to the breath and developing a deeper connection between the mind and body. This calm focus can help reduce stress and promote mental clarity, making it an excellent pose to start or end a yoga practice. For beginners, learning to stand tall and breathe deeply in Mountain Pose can be a gateway to experiencing the transformative effects of yoga, both physically and mentally.

In Short

'Tadasana' is a Sanskrit term made up of two words where 'tada' implies 'palm' or 'mountain' and 'asana' signifies 'posture' or 'seat'. The Tadasana posture is the physical embodiment of standing strong like a tree or a vast mountain. Hence, it is also called the Mountain pose or palm tree stance.

Benefits: Improves posture, strengthens legs, and promotes balance.

How to do: Stand tall with feet together, arms at sides. Ground your feet, engage your thighs, and lengthen through the spine.

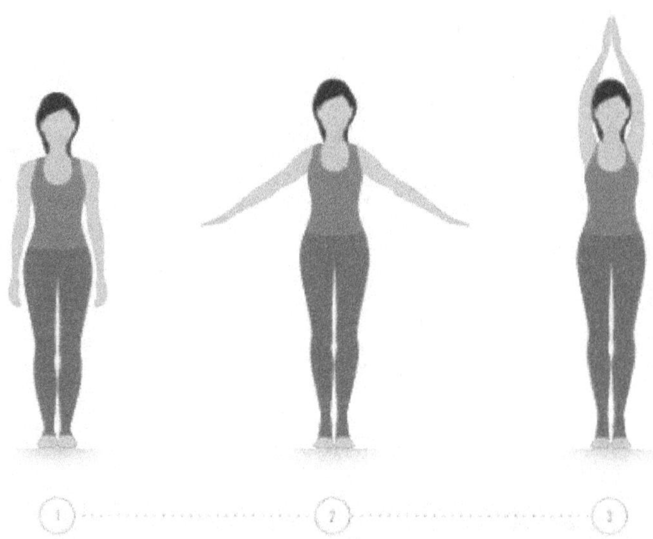

Chapter 2

Downward-Facing Dog (Adho Mukha Svanasana)

Downward-Facing Dog (Adho Mukha Svanasana) is one of the most recognized and widely practiced yoga poses, especially for beginners, due to its powerful benefits for both the body and mind. This inverted "V" shaped posture serves as a full-body stretch, engaging muscles from the arms and shoulders to the legs and feet. To begin, start on your hands and knees in a tabletop position. Place your hands shoulder-width apart and spread your fingers, pressing firmly into the mat. Curl your toes under, and as you exhale, lift your hips toward the ceiling, straightening your legs while keeping a slight bend in the knees if necessary.

One of the primary benefits of Downward-Facing Dog is that it stretches the entire back body—hamstrings, calves, spine, and shoulders—while strengthening the arms and legs. The pose creates length through the spine, which can help to alleviate back pain caused by sitting for long periods or poor posture. The active engagement of your hands, arms, and shoulders provides strength and stability, helping to tone and condition these areas over time. For beginners, it's important not to focus on having perfectly straight legs, but rather on finding alignment and comfort in the pose. With regular practice, flexibility will improve.

In addition to its physical benefits, Downward-Facing Dog is a grounding pose that helps to center and focus the mind. As an inversion, it shifts your perspective by having your heart above your head, encouraging blood flow to the brain. This increased circulation can bring a sense of mental clarity and rejuvenation. Practicing deep, steady breathing in this position calms the nervous system and promotes relaxation, making it a wonderful pose for stress relief. By focusing on the breath, you also learn to quiet the mind, helping you cultivate mindfulness and reduce anxiety.

This pose can serve as a transitional or resting posture in many yoga sequences, providing an opportunity to reconnect with your breath and regain energy before moving into more challenging poses. For beginners, Downward Dog may initially feel intense, especially if the hamstrings or shoulders are tight. However, with practice, it becomes a resting posture where you can settle in and rejuvenate the body. The sensation of grounding your hands into the mat and stretching your body towards the sky symbolizes a balance between effort and relaxation.

Mentally, Downward-Facing Dog teaches patience and perseverance. It can feel challenging at first, but with consistent practice, it becomes more comfortable and even meditative. As you hold the pose, you learn to focus on alignment, breath, and balance, which helps to quiet distractions and center your mind. This combination of physical effort and mental stillness makes Downward Dog not only a key posture in yoga but also a valuable tool for overall well-being, cultivating both strength and serenity.

In Short

Benefits: Strengthens arms and legs, stretches the back, shoulders, and hamstrings.

How to do: Start on your hands and knees, then lift your hips up and back, creating an inverted "V" shape with your body.

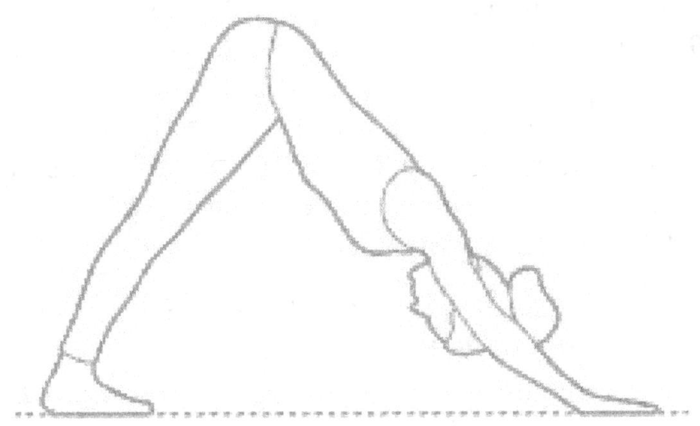

Chapter 3

Child's Pose (Balasana)

Child's Pose (Balasana) is a gentle and restorative yoga posture that provides numerous benefits for both the body and mind. It's often used as a resting pose in yoga sequences, allowing practitioners to pause, reconnect with their breath, and release tension. To get into the pose, start by kneeling on the floor with your big toes touching and your knees either together or slightly apart. Sit back on your heels, then exhale as you fold forward, bringing your chest towards your thighs and extending your arms in front of you, with your forehead resting on the mat. If this feels too intense, you can modify by placing a blanket or cushion between your thighs and calves, or rest your forehead on a block for added support.

One of the primary benefits of Child's Pose is that it provides a deep stretch to the back, hips, and thighs. By folding forward, you gently stretch and lengthen the spine, helping to alleviate tension in the lower back and neck. This is particularly beneficial for people who spend long hours sitting or standing, as it helps to release the compression in the spine. Additionally, the pose stretches the hips, knees, and ankles, promoting flexibility in these joints. Because the pose is passive, it allows the muscles to relax deeply, making it an effective way to release physical tension.

Beyond its physical benefits, Child's Pose is also incredibly calming for the mind. It is a naturally grounding and inward-focused posture, helping to calm the nervous system and reduce stress. The gentle forward fold combined with deep, steady breathing activates the parasympathetic nervous system, which promotes relaxation and rest. As you fold into yourself, the pose creates a sense of safety and comfort, helping to ease anxiety and soothe the mind. It's often referred to as a "comfort pose" because of the way it nurtures and supports both body and mind during moments of overwhelm or fatigue.

Child's Pose is also a valuable tool for cultivating mindfulness. Since the posture is restorative and requires minimal physical effort, it allows you to focus on your breath and develop a deeper connection between the body and mind. Practicing slow, deliberate breathing while in the pose helps you become more aware of your body and any areas of tension or discomfort. This mindfulness not only enhances your yoga practice but can also carry over into your daily life, helping you stay present and grounded in the moment.

For beginners, Child's Pose offers an accessible way to find rest and relief during a yoga practice. It's a posture that invites you to listen to your body and honor your limits, making it an ideal pose for those new to yoga. Whether used as a transition between more challenging poses or as a moment of stillness at the end of a practice, Child's Pose offers deep physical and mental benefits, helping to restore balance, relieve stress, and promote overall well-being.

In Short

Benefits: Stretches the hips, thighs, and ankles while calming the mind.

How to do: Kneel on the floor, sit back on your heels, and stretch your arms forward with your forehead resting on the mat.

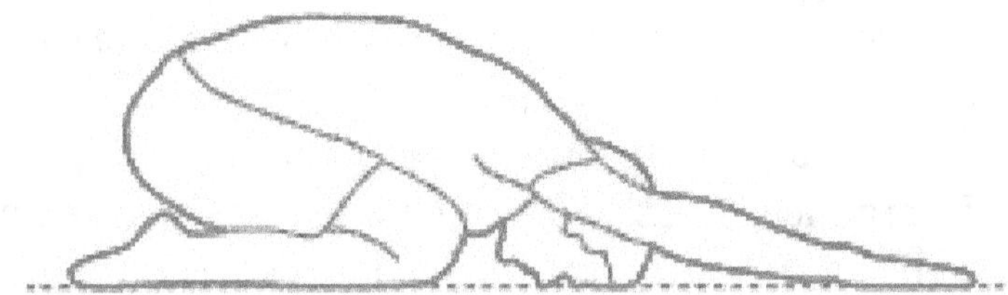

Chapter 4

Cat-Cow Pose (Marjaryasana/ Bitilasana)

Cat-Cow Pose (Marjaryasana/Bitilasana) is a dynamic, flowing yoga sequence that combines two complementary poses to promote spinal flexibility and mindful movement. This gentle back-and-forth motion between Cat Pose (Marjaryasana) and Cow Pose (Bitilasana) is often used as a warm-up in yoga practice to loosen up the spine, improve posture, and bring awareness to the breath. To begin, start on your hands and knees in a tabletop position with your wrists aligned under your shoulders and your knees under your hips. As you inhale, drop
your belly toward the mat, lift your chest, and look upward into Cow Pose, allowing the spine to arch gently. On the exhale, round your back, tucking your chin toward your chest and pulling your belly button toward your spine, flowing into Cat Pose.

The primary benefit of Cat-Cow Pose is its ability to increase flexibility and mobility in the spine. By alternating between arching and rounding the back, you stretch and strengthen the muscles surrounding the spine, which can help alleviate stiffness and improve posture. This is especially beneficial for people who experience back pain due to poor posture or long hours of sitting. The gentle spinal movement encourages the natural range of motion, lubricating the vertebrae and improving circulation to the spinal discs, which can reduce discomfort and prevent injury over time.

Beyond its spinal benefits, Cat-Cow Pose also helps to open up the chest, shoulders, and hips. The stretching of the chest and shoulders in Cow Pose creates space and can improve respiratory function by encouraging deeper, fuller breaths. In Cat Pose, the rounding of the spine and drawing in of the belly engages the core muscles, providing a gentle abdominal workout while also massaging the organs, which can aid digestion. The gentle flow between these two poses also helps to release tension in the neck and lower back, making it a great practice for overall body relaxation and release.

Mentally, Cat-Cow Pose is an excellent way to bring mindfulness into your yoga practice. The rhythmic coordination of movement with the breath encourages a deeper connection between the body and mind, fostering present-moment awareness. As you move slowly and intentionally through the poses, you cultivate focus and relaxation, which can help reduce stress and anxiety. By focusing on the breath, you also learn to regulate your breathing, which promotes calmness and helps manage tension or mental fatigue. This flowing sequence acts as a moving meditation, allowing the mind to quiet and the body to release built-up stress.

For beginners, Cat-Cow Pose is an accessible and gentle way to ease into more challenging yoga postures. It can be practiced by anyone, regardless of flexibility, and serves as a foundational movement for spinal health and breath awareness. The pose's ability to soothe both the body and mind makes it ideal for transitioning into a yoga session or for moments when you need to reconnect with yourself. By regularly practicing Cat-Cow, you can improve your physical posture, enhance your mental clarity, and develop a deeper sense of balance between your mind and body.

In Short

Benefits: Increases flexibility in the spine and stretches the back.
How to do: On your hands and knees, alternate between arching your back (Cow) and rounding your back (Cat).

Cat

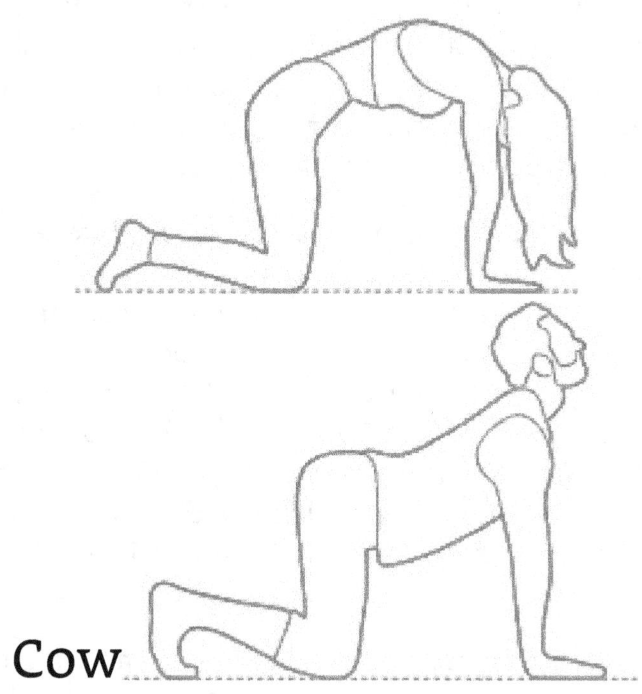

Chapter 5

Warrior I (Virabhadrasana I)

Warrior I (Virabhadrasana I) is a powerful standing yoga pose that builds strength, stability, and focus. It is often used in yoga sequences to cultivate endurance and balance while also providing a deep stretch to various parts of the body. To execute the pose, start from a standing position and step one foot back, keeping the front knee bent at a 90-degree angle and the back leg straight. Square your hips toward the front of the mat, raise your arms overhead with palms facing each other, and ground both feet firmly into the floor. As you hold the pose, keep your core engaged and lengthen your spine, creating a strong, stable base while reaching upward through your fingertips.

Physically, Warrior I strengthens the legs, glutes, and core muscles, while also stretching the hips, chest, and shoulders. The deep lunge engages and tones the quadriceps, hamstrings, and calves, building lower body strength and endurance. At the same time, the pose encourages flexibility in the hip flexors and groin, making it especially beneficial for individuals who experience tightness in these areas from prolonged sitting. The raised arms and open chest also help stretch the shoulders and upper body, promoting better posture and relieving tension in the back and neck.

Warrior I also promotes body alignment and balance, as it requires both strength and coordination to maintain the pose. Squaring the hips and shoulders toward the front while maintaining stability in the legs helps improve overall body awareness and alignment. Over time, practicing this pose can enhance balance and stability, both on and off the mat. Additionally, by grounding the feet firmly into the mat and extending through the spine, Warrior I creates a strong connection between the body and the earth, fostering a sense of rootedness and stability.

Mentally, Warrior I symbolizes focus, determination, and inner strength. Holding the pose requires concentration, which helps train the mind to stay present and focused. As you balance the effort in your legs with the lengthening of your upper body, you cultivate a sense of calm and perseverance, even in the face of physical challenge. This mental discipline carries over into daily life, helping you manage stress and distractions with greater ease. By focusing on your breath while holding the pose, you can also tap into a sense of mindfulness, calming the mind and reducing anxiety.

Warrior I is not only a physically empowering pose but also a mentally invigorating one. For beginners, it provides an opportunity to build both strength and flexibility while practicing focus and balance. The pose's combination of physical engagement and mental steadiness makes it a key posture for cultivating resilience, body awareness, and clarity of mind. As you continue to practice Warrior I, you'll develop greater stamina, both in your body and in your ability to face challenges with grace and strength.

In Short

Benefits: Strengthens legs and shoulders, stretches the hips and chest.

How to do: Step one foot back and bend the front knee while raising your arms overhead.

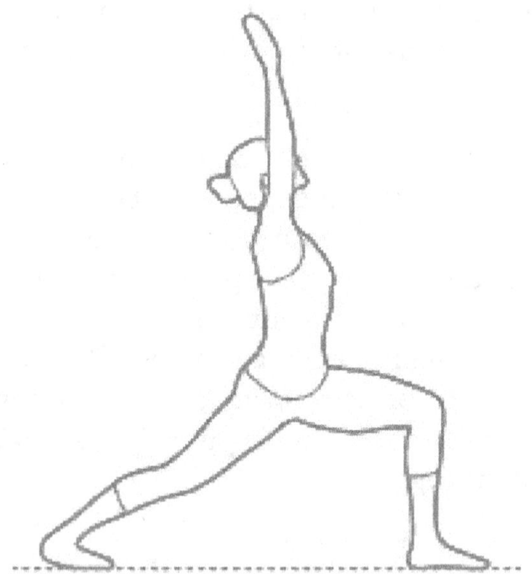

Chapter 6

Warrior II (Virabhadrasana II)

Warrior II (Virabhadrasana II) is a foundational yoga pose that emphasizes strength, stability, and focus. It is a powerful stance that opens the hips, stretches the legs, and engages the arms and shoulders. To practice Warrior II, start in a standing position and step one foot back, turning the back foot out slightly and aligning the heel with the front foot. Bend the front knee to a 90-degree angle, keeping the knee over the ankle, and extend your arms parallel to the ground, palms facing down. Your torso should remain upright, and your gaze is directed forward over the front hand, cultivating a sense of focus and determination.

Physically, Warrior II strengthens the legs, hips, and shoulders, making it a key pose for building endurance and stability. The deep bend in the front knee engages the quadriceps and glutes, while the back leg remains strong and grounded, stretching the inner thighs and hip flexors. The extended arms and active engagement of the shoulder muscles help build upper body strength and improve posture. The pose also promotes greater flexibility in the hips, groin, and chest.
Regular practice of Warrior II can improve lower body stability and stamina, which can enhance athletic performance and overall mobility.

One of the most significant aspects of Warrior II is its focus on alignment and balance. The pose requires the hips to open while keeping the torso aligned with the legs, which helps develop body awareness and coordination. This focus on alignment strengthens the core muscles as they work to keep the body stable and upright. Warrior II encourages practitioners to find strength and balance between effort and ease, teaching the body to remain grounded while reaching out with energy through the arms. This balance of stability and expansion improves overall body control and encourages greater symmetry in movement.

Mentally, Warrior II is a pose of focus, determination, and inner strength. As you hold the position, you cultivate a sense of mental clarity and resilience. The pose's grounding nature fosters a connection to the earth, helping you feel more stable and centered. Focusing your gaze over the front hand, known as your "drishti," allows you to practice concentration and mindfulness. By holding the pose and breathing deeply, you can train your mind to remain calm and focused, even when faced with physical challenges. This mental discipline not only enhances your yoga practice but also helps you manage stress and distractions in daily life.

Warrior II also symbolizes a warrior's spirit of perseverance and inner power. For beginners, this pose teaches patience and focus, as it requires sustained effort and balance. By holding Warrior II for several breaths, you learn to maintain your strength while remaining calm and composed, both physically and mentally. The combination of strength, balance, and focus in Warrior II makes it an essential posture for developing both physical endurance and mental resilience.

Over time, practicing this pose can lead to greater confidence, inner strength, and the ability to stay grounded in the present moment, both on and off the mat.

In Short

Benefits: Enhances strength and endurance in the legs, opens the hips, and stretches the arms and shoulders.

How to do: From a standing position, step one foot back, bend the front knee, and stretch your arms out to the sides.

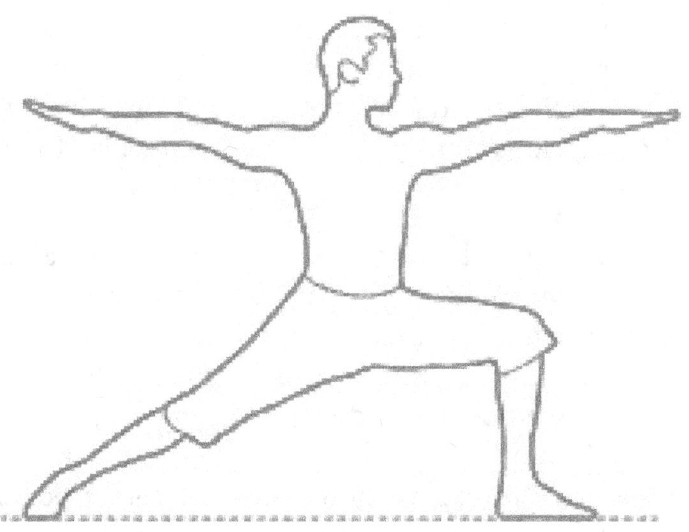

Chapter 7

Tree Pose (Vrksasana)

Tree Pose (Vrksasana) is a balancing yoga posture that promotes stability, focus, and a sense of grounding. It's one of the most accessible standing balance poses, making it a great option for beginners. To perform Tree Pose, begin by standing tall in Mountain Pose (Tadasana). Shift your weight onto one foot, rooting firmly into the ground, and slowly lift the opposite foot. Place the sole of your lifted foot on the inner thigh, calf, or ankle of the standing leg—just avoid placing it on the knee joint. Bring your palms together at your chest or extend your arms overhead like branches. Hold your gaze steady on a fixed point to maintain balance.

Physically, Tree Pose is excellent for improving balance and strengthening the muscles in the legs and core. The act of standing on one leg requires engagement from the stabilizing muscles in the ankles, calves, thighs, and hips. Over time, this strengthens your legs and improves your overall sense of stability. Additionally, holding your arms overhead stretches the shoulders and upper body, promoting better posture and alignment. Tree Pose also encourages flexibility in the hips, as it requires you to open your hip joint to place the lifted foot. For beginners, it's important to start with the foot lower on the leg, gradually increasing the challenge as balance improves.

Beyond its physical benefits, Tree Pose is powerful for cultivating mental focus and clarity. To maintain balance in the pose, it's essential to focus your gaze on a single point in front of you (called a "drishti"). This practice of concentration helps quiet the mind and keeps you anchored in the present moment. Balancing postures like Tree Pose challenge your ability to stay calm and composed, even when you feel off balance. By practicing this regularly, you strengthen your mental focus, which can carry over into other areas of life, helping you handle distractions or stress with more ease.

Tree Pose is also a pose that fosters a sense of grounding and connection to the earth. As you root your standing foot into the ground, you create a stable foundation that symbolizes being grounded in your own strength and stability. The pose encourages you to find balance between effort and relaxation, teaching you to stay strong yet flexible. This grounding quality can be incredibly calming, especially during moments of stress or anxiety, helping you feel more connected and centered.

For beginners, Tree Pose serves as a great introduction to balance work in yoga, while offering the opportunity to develop both physical strength and mental resilience. It encourages patience, as balance improves over time with practice. By focusing on alignment, breath, and a steady gaze, Tree Pose becomes not just a physical exercise but a meditative one as well. The dual benefit of enhancing balance in the body and stillness in the mind makes Tree Pose a valuable tool for overall well-being and inner stability, both on and off the mat.

In Short

Benefits: Improves balance, strengthens legs, and opens the hips.
How to do: Stand on one leg, place the opposite foot on the inner thigh or calf, and bring your hands together at your chest or overhead.

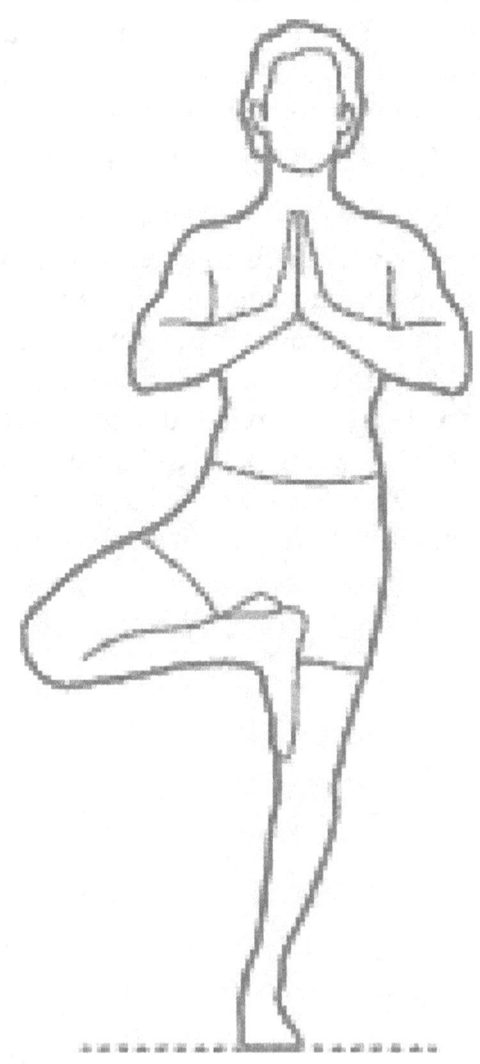

Chapter 8

Bridge Pose (Setu Bandhasana)

Bridge Pose (Setu Bandhasana) is a foundational backbend in yoga that offers significant benefits for both the body and mind. It is an accessible pose for beginners and can be used to build strength, improve flexibility, and promote relaxation. To perform Bridge Pose, lie on your back with your knees bent and feet flat on the ground, hip-width apart. Place your arms alongside your body, palms facing down. As you inhale, press your feet and arms into the mat and lift your hips toward the ceiling, creating a bridge shape with your body. Engage your glutes and thighs while keeping your knees parallel and your chest lifted toward your chin.

Physically, Bridge Pose strengthens several key muscle groups, including the glutes, hamstrings, and lower back. The lifting of the hips engages the muscles in the lower body, while the action of pressing your arms and shoulders into the mat helps build upper body strength.
This pose also stretches the chest, neck, spine, and hip flexors, making it an effective counterbalance to the slouched posture many people develop from prolonged sitting or working at a desk. Practicing Bridge Pose regularly can help open the chest and shoulders, improving posture and relieving tension in the back and neck.

In addition to its strength-building and flexibility-enhancing qualities, Bridge Pose is also beneficial for spinal health. The gentle backbend helps to realign the spine, promoting flexibility and mobility. By lifting the hips and creating a gentle curve in the back, Bridge Pose encourages space between the vertebrae, which can relieve compression in the spine and help alleviate lower back pain. This pose also stimulates the abdominal organs, improving digestion and circulation, while the gentle inversion (as your heart is slightly above your head) boosts blood flow to the brain, promoting mental clarity.

Mentally, Bridge Pose can have a calming and grounding effect on the mind. As you hold the posture and focus on your breath, it encourages a deep sense of relaxation. The pose helps activate the parasympathetic nervous system, which is responsible for the body's
rest-and-digest response. This activation helps reduce stress, lower anxiety, and promote a sense of calm. The heart-opening aspect of the pose can also have emotional benefits, as it invites a feeling of openness and vulnerability, which can help release pent-up emotions or tension.

For beginners, Bridge Pose is a great way to gently explore backbends and experience the benefits of opening the chest and strengthening the core and lower body. The pose encourages you to focus on alignment and breath, fostering both physical and mental awareness. As you press into the ground and lift your body, you cultivate a sense of grounding and stability, while the gentle stretch helps release tension and stress. This combination of physical strength, flexibility, and mental relaxation makes Bridge Pose a valuable tool for enhancing overall
well-being, promoting spinal health, and creating a deep sense of inner calm.

In Short

Benefits: Strengthens the back, glutes, and hamstrings while stretching the chest and spine. **How to do**: Lie on your back, bend your knees, and lift your hips toward the ceiling while pressing your feet into the floor.

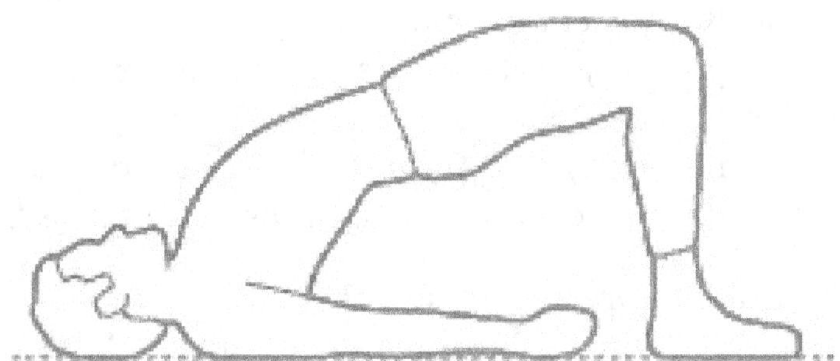

Chapter 9

Seated Forward Bend
(Paschimottanasana)

Seated Forward Bend (Paschimottanasana) is a calming and restorative yoga posture that emphasizes flexibility, relaxation, and introspection. It is often practiced at the end of a yoga sequence to promote relaxation and prepare the body for meditation or rest. To perform Seated Forward Bend, start by sitting on the floor with your legs extended straight in front of you. Flex your feet, keeping your heels grounded, and engage your thighs to protect your knees. As you inhale, lengthen your spine, reaching your arms overhead. On your exhale, hinge at your hips and gently fold forward, reaching for your feet, ankles, or shins while keeping your spine as long as possible.

Physically, Seated Forward Bend offers a deep stretch to the entire posterior chain of the body, including the hamstrings, calves, and lower back. This pose helps to improve flexibility in the hamstrings, which is essential for overall mobility and can reduce the risk of injury, particularly for those who engage in activities that require leg strength and flexibility. The gentle stretching of the lower back and spine also helps alleviate tension and stiffness, making it a great remedy for discomfort caused by prolonged sitting or standing. Additionally, as you fold forward, the position encourages relaxation in the hips and pelvis, further enhancing flexibility in this area.

In terms of spinal health, Seated Forward Bend promotes lengthening and decompression of the vertebrae. By bending forward, you create space in the lumbar region of the spine, which can relieve compression and improve circulation to the spinal discs. This gentle forward fold also encourages better posture, as it reinforces awareness of spinal alignment. Regular practice of Seated Forward Bend can enhance overall body awareness and alignment, promoting a healthier spine and reducing the risk of chronic back pain.

Mentally, Seated Forward Bend fosters a sense of calm and introspection. As you move into the pose and focus on your breath, you naturally shift your attention inward, allowing for a moment of reflection and mindfulness. The forward bend can help ease anxiety and stress by activating the parasympathetic nervous system, which encourages relaxation and a sense of grounding.
Holding the pose for several breaths provides an opportunity to practice mindfulness, cultivating a deeper connection to your body and breath while letting go of distractions.

For beginners, Seated Forward Bend is a valuable pose for exploring flexibility and developing a mindful yoga practice. It encourages patience and self-acceptance, as everyone has different levels of flexibility and comfort in the pose. If reaching for the feet feels challenging, beginners can use a strap or simply rest their hands on their shins. This adaptability allows practitioners to enjoy the benefits of the pose while honoring their bodies. Overall, Seated Forward Bend is a gentle yet impactful pose that promotes physical flexibility, spinal health, and mental calmness, making it an essential component of any yoga practice.

In Short

Benefits: Stretches the spine, hamstrings, and lower back.
How to do: Sit with your legs extended in front of you, hinge at the hips, and reach for your toes.

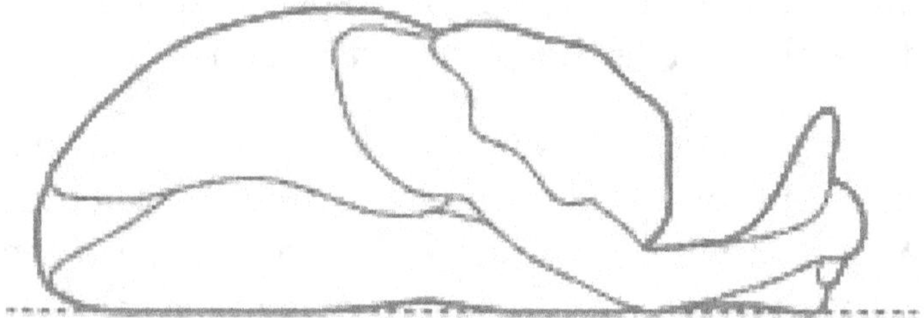

Chapter 10

Corpse Pose (Savasana)

Corpse Pose (Savasana) is often regarded as one of the most essential poses in yoga, serving as a final resting position that allows practitioners to integrate the benefits of their practice. While it may appear simple, executing Savasana correctly can be a challenge, particularly for beginners who may find it difficult to relax fully. To begin, lie flat on your back with your legs extended comfortably apart, allowing your feet to naturally fall open. Your arms should be positioned alongside your body, palms facing upward, and your head aligned with your spine. Close your eyes and take a few deep breaths, allowing your body to sink into the ground. Focus on letting go of any tension in your muscles and releasing any thoughts or distractions.

Physically, Corpse Pose provides a wealth of benefits for the body. It encourages complete relaxation, which can help lower blood pressure and reduce stress levels. As the body settles into stillness, it allows for the muscles to recover and rejuvenate after a yoga practice.
Savasana also aids in restoring energy, as it promotes deep relaxation that can relieve tension in both the body and mind. By calming the nervous system, Corpse Pose can enhance overall well-being, making it a critical component of any yoga session.

On a mental level, Savasana is a powerful practice in mindfulness and meditation. As you lie still, the focus shifts inward, inviting a sense of tranquility and awareness. This pose encourages you to observe your thoughts and feelings without judgment, cultivating a sense of presence and acceptance. It allows the mind to slow down and creates a space for reflection and introspection. This practice of letting go of mental clutter can lead to reduced anxiety and improved emotional balance, enhancing your overall mental health.

For beginners, it's essential to approach Corpse Pose with an open mind and a willingness to embrace stillness. If you find it challenging to relax, consider using props such as a bolster or blanket to support your body. Placing a pillow under your knees can help relieve lower back tension, while covering yourself with a light blanket can create a sense of security. Focus on your breath, allowing it to guide you into a deeper state of relaxation. If your mind begins to wander, gently bring your attention back to your breath or the sensations in your body.

Ultimately, Corpse Pose is not just a resting position but a vital practice that promotes integration and mindfulness. It invites a moment of stillness where the benefits of your yoga practice can be fully absorbed. For beginners, mastering Savasana can enhance their overall experience in yoga, teaching the importance of rest and reflection. By incorporating this pose into your routine, you'll cultivate a deeper connection to your body and mind, fostering a sense of peace and well-being that extends beyond the yoga mat.

In Short

Benefits: Promotes relaxation and stress relief.

How to do: Lie flat on your back with arms at your sides, legs relaxed, and breathe deeply.

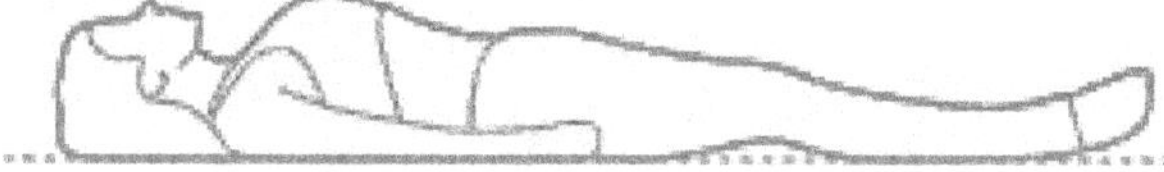

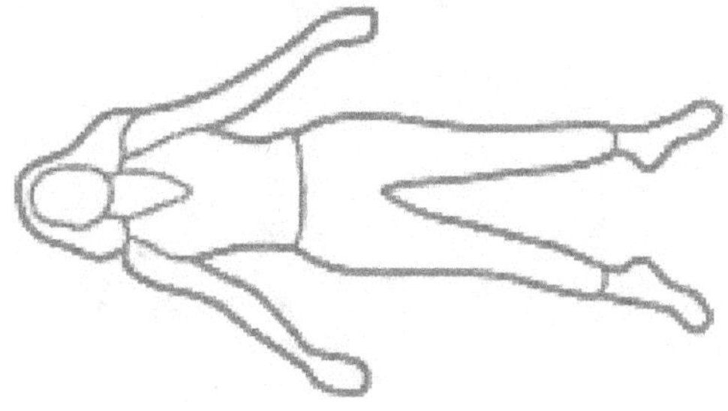